Intermittent Fasting 16/8

*How to Effortlessly Improve Health,
Control Hunger, Lose Weight, and
Slow Down Aging While Still Enjoying
Life and Your Favorite Foods*

Rebekah Addams

Table of Contents

Introduction

Health and fitness are two things, usually synonymous, that are becoming more and more far-fetched for those people around the world who aren't affected by their outward appearance or sluggish nature or are "too busy" to make time for exercise. Being healthy doesn't mean 'stick thin' or bulging muscles, it means any excess weight is maintained and staying on top of nutrition all while feeling good about what you see in the mirror.

It might look simple laid out in a sentence, but for most, this is not a reality. People of all ages have come to rely on unrealistic fad diets and short, quick burst workouts that are greatly unsustainable in the grand scheme of good health. Many diets require you to eat six meals per day, others every three hours, which in turn requires you to meal prep every week. The logic is if you plan your meals ahead of time, you're less likely to binge eat on junk food, or order takeout but this means a lot of preplanning and sacrificing one day each week to spend in the kitchen.

Relying on hard diets and exhaustive workouts to drastically change your life will only provide temporary relief to your struggle. Instead, a lifestyle change that will help you retain your good health and shed weight is a much better alternative. If you truly want to stay healthy and lose weight, intermittent fasting is the way to go.

Though there are many different ways to fast, the 16/8 intermittent method is by far the best of them all. It is flexible, safe, sustainable, and ultimately more doable. When I first struggled with weight loss and staying healthy, I experimented with almost every diet plan available. Many diets required me to split my caloric intake into six or more small meals throughout the day. This meant my meal sizes were basically microscopic, I was never satisfied, and this led to incessant hunger and frequent snacking. Also, my job was structured in a way that I had no real time to squeeze in a meal every three hours. This led to wider gaps between meals that left me 'hangry.' With intermittent fasting, I have larger, sufficient meals that require minimal prep work. My daily caloric intake is divided into the meals that fit into my small eating window. This means I have larger, more satisfying meals that keep me fuller, longer.

Intermittent fasting provides many truly amazing benefits. You have a specific eating window as opposed to eating every three hours giving you a great deal of flexibility within that window. Intermittent fasting allows you to be more productive, have larger, more sustainable meals, save time spent preparing and planning meals, and will also help you save money.

One of the biggest advantages of intermittent fasting is it uses fat to produce energy for the various processes in the body. When your body is freed from having to constantly digest food, it can use saved energy for other useful purposes like healing or cleansing the body of harmful substances. This fat-burning mechanism is what helps you lose weight. According to a study by the

University of Illinois in Chicago, it was found that intermittent fasting, specifically the time-restricted fasting like the 16/8 method was an extremely effective way to achieve weight loss in obese patients. The participants also reported intermittent fasting helping clear their head as well as increase concentration and cognitive abilities.

With this book, I want to provide you a thorough understanding of what intermittent fasting is and how it can truly help you lose weight and stay healthy. Let this be your guide to adopting a new lifestyle; a lifestyle that actually helps you achieve a greater good and delivers on its promise. Here you will be able to calculate your own daily calorie intake and plan your eating window accordingly with my 21-day quick start guide. I have prepared an easy to make, flavorful menu of healthy recipes with nutritional value included that you can choose from, alter, and accommodate your intermittent fasting schedule.

It is common knowledge that the sooner you take control of your health and weight goals the better you will be because it is easier to maintain than to transform. And as you age it only gets harder to maintain control of your health and body. So with this, I urge you to give the 16/8 method of intermittent fasting a try as soon as you finish this book or as you read along. Implement the strategies mentioned here for lasting changes made to you and your quality of life.

Also, if you would like some extra support from me, I would love for you to join my private Facebook group, where you can speak to me directly, ask any questions you might have, and how you can personally apply fasting to your lifestyle and unique needs. I would be honored to help you along this journey, and it will give you a chance to mingle and chat with other people on the same path as you.

Just look up **intermittent fasting, fuel the brain, lose the fat** in the Facebook search bar, send your request to join, answer the three questions and I'll accept you straight away!

I have outlined for my readers a special intermittent fasting cheat sheet which can be used as a valuable tool in ensuring you're on the right track from the very start. This gives you a checklist of the most important aspects of the method. I want you to get the most out of this lifestyle and keep you from making the common mistakes a lot of newbies fall prey to on their first try.

If you are interested in this cheat sheet, go to **www.thefastingfacts.com** Enter your details and I will send them straight to your inbox

Chapter 1: Intermittent Fasting and the 16/8 Method

Intermittent fasting is a method by which your body burns stored fats and morphs it into a self-cleaning machine. The fat burning will make you lose excess weight and cleansing will help to restore any injured or broken cells as well as repair tissue in the body, all while getting rid of lingering and harmful substances. This occurs employing a controlled and timed eating schedule. Intermittent fasting has many different methods but each works using the same basic principle. Someone who is fasting abstains from any food for a fixed period and eats within a specific range of time known as the eating window. The fasting period could be a few hours with a minimum fasting range of 12 to even 24 hours. Some fasting mechanisms require fasting for days together with nothing but water to drink. But out of all these methods, the most suitable method for people of a wide age group is the 16/8 method.

The 16/8 Method

The 16/8 method is the most practical with a fasting period of sixteen hours and an eating window of eight hours. It sets the right balance between the fasting and feeding to give your body sufficient time to burn excess fats and cleanse the body safely without straining itself too much. For both beginners and seasoned practitioners of intermittent fasting, 16/8 is an ideal way to stay healthy. Intermittent fasting is not a diet plan with restrictions on what to eat or what to avoid. Instead, it is a lifestyle that tells you when to eat rather than what to eat making this method more sustainable in the long run.

The Two States of Our Body

Our body is always in either of the two natural states. A feeding state and a fasting state. When we eat, our body goes into a feeding state and remains in this state for about 4 to 5 hours. The important thing with this state is we do not feel hungry when in a feeding state. Our body is busy making use of the meal we have just had to obtain energy from it. The food is digested and sugars are produced. These sugars are used to generate enough energy for our functions. After the feeding state for about eight hours or so comes the post-feeding state. This is also known as the intermediate stage where we may or may not feel hungry. Then the fasting state that lasts until our next meal. Our body has used up the last meal's digested sugars for energy and in this fasting state, if and when our body needs energy it will turn to stored energy reserves as fuel. This stored energy is nothing but stored fat. So, that means, the longer the fasting state, the more fat that is burned to produce energy to sustain our bodies.

Intermittent fasting, of whatever kind, aims to make optimum use of this fasting state to burn excess fats and kick start the cleansing process. Some programs have periods of over 24 hours, meaning the body has a prolonged fasting state. But this isn't ideal for everyone as it can be quite challenging for a fasting newbie to attempt.

Instead, adopting something flexible with only 16 hours of fasting is far easier and extremely doable with practice.

The Science Behind Intermittent Fasting

So, how does intermittent fasting work? What happens in our bodies that leads to the burning of fats and cleansing processes to occur when we fast? Understanding this is essential to get the right picture of intermittent fasting and make the system work to our advantage.

When we eat or drink, our bodies produce insulin. It is a hormone that regulates the levels of sugar or glucose in our blood. Whatever is ingested gets converted into usable forms of sugar as glucose. The sugars that aren't needed right away are stored in the form of glycogen, which is nothing but a ready-to-use form of glucose. Whatever else remains, gets converted into fats and is stored up for later use. All these processes are conducted under the supervision of our very own insulin! This is the reason why it is also termed as the fat-storing hormone.

In the absence of insulin, the production and efficient storage of sugars take a back seat and this is why people with type 2 diabetes need supplemental insulin injections to control their sugar levels because their bodies are unable to naturally produce insulin. When we are eating regularly then our body is doing the same with insulin production. This results in regular fat stores in our body because we don't need that much glucose to function normally. So, the more you eat, the more insulin is being produced creating or filling fat deposits. Regulating our insulin levels is the key to control weight gain. Insulin plays a vital role, but at the right time and in the right amounts.

Two other hormones play an important role in our body's response to food. These are ghrelin and leptin. Ghrelin is a hunger hormone, which means it signals us when we are hungry and need to eat. But the problem with ghrelin is not all of its hunger signals are true. Consider this: From an early age we are conditioned to eat three times a day. Breakfast, lunch, and dinner is as natural a routine as breathing. We need not necessarily feel hungry at each mealtime, but because our body has been taught to expect/receive food at these hours, it signals to us that we are hungry. Ghrelin hormone is released at these mealtimes which tells us we need to eat even if our body is still in a feeding state from our last meal.

Leptin is a satiety hormone. It signals when we have had enough food and need to stop. It is an important hormone that regulates our food intake and in turn, is responsible for how much of that food gets stored as fat. Right from the time we are born, our bodies are in sync with our nutritional needs and these hormones are in a perfect balance. But as we grow and adapt to unhealthy eating practices, this balance is broken and we tend to eat more and store more.

This is where intermittent fasting comes into play. It regulates hormone levels and directs our body to make use of fat stores for energy. In the fasting state, there is no food therefore no insulin to store fat. Instead, when we tap into our fat stores for energy, we are signaling our body that we have enough at our disposal and do not need more food. This regulates the levels and release times of both ghrelin and leptin.

Benefits of 16/8 Intermittent Fasting Method

Intermittent fasting has numerous benefits. The 16/8 method, in particular, has a lot of advantages in addition to being the simplest, safest, and the most doable method of all the different intermittent fasting methods. Let's see a few of these benefits below.

Fat Burn/Weight Loss

One of the biggest advantages of any intermittent fasting technique is the assurance of weight loss through fat burn. No other diets that promise weight loss can deliver with such an assurance for a long and permanent duration. Because intermittent fasting is a lifestyle change and not a random diet restriction this should assure you that the fat burn is long-lasting and permanent.

This is a guaranteed result because the science behind it is flawless and anyone practicing intermittent fasting will see the results of being in an extended fasted state are efficient weight loss and fat burn. When the body's immediate reserves of glucose are depleted, it moves on to ready to use glucose stored as glycogen. When these are exhausted, the body moves on to consuming the fat stores to produce energy. This fat burning process is known as ketosis, which produces ketones which are a signal of the fat-burning process. A body in a prolonged fasting state shows the presence of ketones in the bloodstream which means the body is actively burning fats. This is a sign to rejoice because the stored fats are at last getting burned. This is what causes weight loss. With any intermittent fasting technique, this is a foolproof process. Though the time of ketosis varies from one method to another based on the number of hours the body spends fasting, all methods have a fat-burning period.

Blood Sugar Regulation

Intermittent fasting also helps regulate the levels of glucose in the blood. As insulin levels gradually decrease as the body moves into the fasting state, the levels of glucose in the bloodstream have already been taken care of. In the fasting state, there is no food, so no insulin and no new glucose is produced. This fasting state gives time to the body to adjust its responses to food and glucose production, with appropriate insulin release in the feeding state. A person with a normal eating schedule eats several meals, big and small, with numerous snacks throughout the day. This means there is always some amount of glucose present in the bloodstream, and several insulin spikes as the day goes on. This is effectively dealt with by fasting.

Boosts Focus and Cognition

Intermittent fasting helps boost brain function. It gives us a special type of mental clarity and improves focus. This happens because a simple 16-hour fast pushes our body into the ketosis process where the body produces ketones and breaks them down to generate energy in place of glucose. It has been known that when the brain uses ketones for energy instead of glucose it gives a boost to the brain's functionality. Also, the hunger hormone ghrelin undergoes a lot of changes during the fasting period. This positively influences the levels of dopamine. Dopamine is a neurotransmitter that is essential for mental clarity and lucid brain function. This is why fasting is said to have a positive effect on how well our brain functions. Our concentration, focus, and cognition is seen to improve by leaps and bounds through intermittent fasting.

Body Cleansing and Longevity

Studies have shown that switching from glucose driven energy processes to ketone-based energy processes causes the body to remain in a cleansing state. The body, when in a fasting period, moves to heal, rectify, restore, and replenish several of its broken and damaged tissues. This helps the body to remain healthy for longer durations. This cleansing also helps remove harmful substances from the body like toxins, waste and broken cells. Also, intermittent fasting has been shown to have several positive effects on keeping diseases at bay, including cancer and Alzheimers.

Stress Resistance

Intermittent fasting also increases our body's resistance to stress of different kinds. Here again, the process of ketosis plays a part. Our body produces a stress-induced hormone known as cortisol. It is necessary to have balanced and low levels of this hormone. Intermittent fasting for longer durations of time with longer fasting periods increases the levels of cortisol in our body and induces greater stress. But, intermittent fasting with gradually increasing fasting periods can actually help regulate cortisol levels and keep stress at bay. This is especially true in the case of the 16/8 method as this has a shorter fasting period compared to other more complex techniques. Methods like OMAD or one meal a day and alternate fasting with twenty-four-hour fasting periods can actually increase stress levels with increased cortisol levels. The opposite is true with the 16/8 method.

Drawbacks of 16/8 Method of Intermittent Fasting

One of the biggest drawbacks of this method of intermittent fasting is the shorter fat-burning period. In a typical sixteen hour fast, the body begins the process of ketosis by the thirteenth hour. So, for a sixteen-hour fast, your body only has three hours to burn fat. Three hours of ketosis results in mild fat consumption. This process occurs at the liver where ketones are produced and is helpful for those suffering from the effects of a fatty liver. Three hours can seem like a short time to effectively carry out the process, but this can be corrected by pushing the body into ketosis quicker. We will discuss this more in-depth in a later chapter.

Chapter 2: Breakfast Is Not the Most Important Meal of the Day

For a long time, we have been told that breakfast is the most important meal of the day. There are several parts of the medical world that propagate this belief and insist on regular breakfast intake, and treat skipping breakfast as a foolish act against good health. But it has been proven that breakfast is not such an important meal after all. Let's look at a couple of reasons that support this theory.

For Weight Loss

When we wake up in the morning, we are in a fasted state, hence the name of the first meal we have after waking up is 'breakfast.' Because essentially, we are breaking our fasts through this meal. But extending this night long fast, farther into the day, is helpful in the long run.

People trying to lose weight are urged to eat a meal, however small, as a breakfast. This is based on the myth that breakfast helps kickstart and speed up your metabolic processes for the day, and your body actively gets into energy producing mode. What is forgotten here is that it actually spikes insulin levels early on in the morning and restricts fat burning. For any weight loss technique to be efficient, you need to burn fat as efficiently as possible. You are already on a fast of at least eight hours or more through the night, making use of these hours and extending to a sixteen hour fast is the ideal way to ensure your fats get burned effectively. Consuming a meal in the morning only defeats the purpose of a night long fast and makes fat burning that much more difficult to achieve.

It is believed that a hearty breakfast leads to reduced appetite throughout the day, and therefore essential for dieters to lose weight and slim down. But intermittent fasting has proven that this is not so. Delaying this meal can actually be the key to losing weight successfully.

For Mental Clarity

It is also believed that breakfast helps improve focus and mental clarity as well as kick starting your metabolism. Instead, extending your overnight fast ensures that less energy is used to digest food and this saved energy can instead be used to improve focus and mental clarity in daily functions. If you think about the origins of man beginning as hunter gatherers, if our environment provided little food for our survival we had to think of new and improved ways to find food or accept the inevitable fate of death thus ending our blood line. So, when you're hungry or fasting you need to be smarter, think more logically and curb that desire for food into more practical use of time. Norepinephrine, the hormone released when fasting and similar to adrenaline, reacts to stress in the body and mobilizes the brain making it prepped and ready for the day ahead. It has shown to improve mental acuity, increase memory retention, and act as blinders for increased focus.

This is not the same case with children and should not be implemented until adulthood. Kids need a well-rounded, healthy breakfast for improved concentration and attention as their bodies are still growing, developing rapidly and require proper nutrition. For adults, conserving energy in any way and putting it to good use can make a difference in the outcome of your day. And all this can make a long-term change in your life by simply extending an overnight fast by a few more hours. Meditate or read the news instead, your body will thank you.

Chapter 3: Increasing Your 16/8 Efficiency

What one type of intermittent fasting offers is more or less the same as the others. But, there are a few elements that are better in some and are lacking in others. Like, in the 16/8 method we see that we have more or less just around three hours to burn fat. This is a short period to burn sufficient amounts of stored fat to tip the scales and see a change in body weight. So, to see this change you need to practice this kind of intermittent fasting for longer durations. There are ways to improve the method's efficiency and you can take steps to ensure significant weight loss occurs in just a matter of days. Below we look at what steps can be taken to help lose weight better while following a 16/8 fasting schedule.

Controlling Insulin

This is a great way to push your body into burning more fat. The logic here is simple. We know that as soon as we eat, we have an insulin spike. As long as we have this insulin in our bloodstream it means we cannot move into fat-burning mode. The sooner the insulin level comes down, the sooner our body can begin utilizing fats.

Remember, insulin is a fat-storing hormone, so its presence hinders burning fat and encourages storage. If we eat something easily digestible, that gives us a relatively smaller insulin spike, it means we will make use of glucose, then the available glycogen, and then move onto stored fats, faster.

So, what can we eat that does not generate a higher insulin spike, is healthy, and also easily digested? Foods that have a lower glycemic index are great at controlling insulin levels. The Glycemic index is food's ability to introduce glucose into the bloodstream. Some foods have a high GI, which means they introduce larger amounts of glucose in the blood while some others with a lower GI produce low amounts. Eating foods with lower GI will ensure lower amounts of glucose in the blood and a lower insulin spike.

This will mean the produced glucose from the digested food will be taken care of quickly, whether by being used as energy or being stored as glycogen. Then the insulin levels will go down gradually and the body can make use of stored energy reserves as available. The sooner this process completes the sooner the body can move to stored fats. Eating proteins along with carbs also helps speed up the process effectively.

Fasted Workouts

We know that our body uses the stored fats to burn and produce energy when in the fasting state. When the body has exhausted all its available glucose and glycogen stores it moves to fats. But, you want your body to burn fat even faster than the natural process. The body will only produce as much energy as it requires. For internal bodily functions, cell work and the like, the body needs energy. But this is not a very high amount, and will not push your body to burn a lot of fat. Only a little fat will be burned to produce what energy is needed. So, what we need to do is to increase the demand we place on our body to supply energy.

One way to do this is to regularly exercise during the fasted state. This is the best strategy to push your body into burning more fats to meet the body's increased energy demands. These exercises could be cardio exercises, yoga, weight training workouts, etc. Simpler exercises like going for walks, stretching, or even dancing and aerobics can make your body burn more fat. Engaging in some form of physical activity will ensure more fat is burned than simply relying on bodily functions or regular routine work to burn sufficient fats.

Timing Workouts and Fast Breaks

If you workout right after you end your eating window, it will not result in fat burn. Timing your workouts correctly to glean as much benefit as possible is also just as essential. Right at the end of your eating window, your body will be high in glucose and glycogen levels. These will be easily used up during your workouts and when you have depleted these two sources, your body will have no reason left to burn excess fats, except for your normal routine or body functions. Which as we now know, doesn't amount to much.

So, time your workouts so that you are ready to break your fast as soon as your workout ends. If you are fasting for sixteen hours, then workout in the last one or two hours before your fast is over and with carbs right after your exercise. This serves two purposes. One, timing your workouts this way ensures you burn sufficient fats. Schedule workouts far from your eating window so there is no chance of glucose or glycogen being used. So, all the energy needed during your workout will be from fats alone. Second, eating carbs right after your workout helps your body make use of glucose needed for muscle building and any repairs. This will, in turn, ensure that any consumed carbs will be used for the muscles and nothing can be stored as fats. Taking care to follow a few simple steps such as these will make sure your 16/8 fast is a lot more fruitful.

Chapter 4: How to Begin Your 16/8 Journey

For someone who has never fasted before, the prospect of going without food for sixteen straight hours can seem daunting and impossible to accomplish. Many enthusiastic intermittent fasters begin their fasting journey with a bang and will fizzle out of both enthusiasm, energy and just can't seem to do it. The reason is their rush to start fasting and seeing results over a few days. Intermittent fasting is indeed fruitful, and it will bring you solid results within a short period. But the key lies in how you ease into the fasting schedule. One might assume that going without food or drinks is easy. They'll jump right into a fasting method and even find the first two days a breeze to accomplish. But on the third day is when reality kicks in and they find themselves wishing to go back to normal eating patterns and leaning toward breaking their fasts midway. What they do not realize, is what sustained them the first two days was simply adrenalin rush and excited enthusiasm. Once that drains off, they are bereft of anything driving their fasts.

Intermittent fasting is not that difficult and need not be that intimidating. What is essential is to gradually ease yourself into the fasting schedules and let your body get used to fasting periods slowly. We will now look at the different steps you can take to start your intermittent fasting journey smoothly and carry on without a hitch.

Correct Mindset

Begin with the right mindset. When you decide to try the 16/8 fasting schedule or any intermittent fasting technique for that matter, prepare yourself mentally first. Be clear about your goals and talk to yourself about what you wish to achieve through this fasting experience. Many times, weight loss simply cannot be achieved by just diet control or exercise. Combining it with the right mindset and intention is the way to begin and finish strong. Diet and exercise will only take you so far. Even if you see results, these will only be temporary as you are not touching on the root cause for weight gain in the first place.

Fat buildup can happen for many different reasons. Fat is stored energy for dire need situations. Beyond this, fats perform other functions too, like offering protection and insulation from the outside world. To understand the reason for this, you might have to look deeper into your mind and look for feelings and thoughts that indicate you are anxious, scared or in fear of something specific. We all have fears and feel threatened from time to time for different reasons we can't always explain. Our body works for us, not against us, and tries to offer some protection with layers of fat because that is its purpose.

The presence of fats might not remove or address your fears, but providing you with these layers is the only way your body can offer external help. It is naturally a psychological issue, and your body cannot address it psychologically, so it does the best it can do by providing you with a layer of protection of fats. The best way to handle such a situation would be to address those fears. Resolve your conflicts and aim to make yourself mentally strong and ready to take on a weight loss challenge.

The next step to correcting and preparing your mindset for effective weight loss before beginning your intermittent fasting schedule is to accept the reality of your situation today. You wish to correct your weight numbers and want to lose the excess fat, but this can only happen when you are at peace with your current self. Make it a point to affirm to yourself that you are happy and love your body and you wish to change to open up to that acceptance even more. Your body will react more positively to your fasting schedules and strategies if you approach it with a positive attitude. All of your fasting times, workouts, and carefully crafted meals will be more effective when you begin with a fresh mind and positive frame of thought.

The Transition of Eating Habits

Once you have readied yourself mentally, then the next step is to slowly transition yourself from your previous lifestyle and eating habits to newer healthier ones. Begin by making note of an average eating day for you. It is a great idea to start a food journal to record your experiences and other occurrences that stand out on your journey with intermittent fasting.

Start by recording your regular eating schedules with your mealtimes. Include any specific snack times you regularly have, any regular drinking like coffee, tea, soda or juice. Also, include any supplements you take on a regular basis. Through all this data you will be able to chart out your plan and schedule your fasting hours to best accommodate your regular needs.

Intermittent fasting will naturally bring a huge change in your eating patterns. But, in the beginning, it is best to keep these changes to a minimum so your transition into fasting is not sudden or abrupt making it easier to handle, both mentally and physically.

Begin your fasts with a twelve-hour fasting period. A twelve-hour fasting period will mean you have the same amount in your eating window. Arrange these eating hours to overlap your regular eating times. It might not accommodate your entire normal eating schedule, but it will help you transition into strict hours of fasting smoother.

Slowly, begin to push back your breakfast to elongate your fasts gradually. Make half an hour increments to your fasts every two to three days. Push back your breakfast regularly and delay it till you reach your sixteen-hour mark.

This slow buildup to the sixteen-hour fast will allow your body to adjust to the rigorous schedule gradually. You will need this adjustment window to let yourself feel at ease with the demands of fasting both physically and emotionally. Continue to journal your experiences as you fast each day. Write down what you feel as your fasting hours go by. Are you excited, hungry, bored, lazy, energetic, or see no change; keep a record of it all. This will help you look back and see what worked and what didn't. Such as which food supported your fasts and which made you hungry sooner; what activities were doable and what seemed stressful? Keeping a record of these little things will strengthen your groundwork as you move along your fasting journey. Also, journaling gives you an outlet for your emotions and will motivate yourself to continue when you feel down physically or in spirit. Personally, my journal was a huge support system on its own for me during my journey of intermittent fasting.

Comfort Foods

Intermittent fasting doesn't really dictate what you eat, it simply tells you when to eat. This, of course, does not mean you eat whatever you like and feel no consequences for your choices. Instead, you need to find the right balance between what is healthy and what is an indulgence. You don't have to give up the comfort food you love, let your favorites be 20 percent of your whole meal plan while eighty percent of caloric intake consists of healthy food. Work out how you would like this to play out. Would you prefer a serving of your favorite every three days or save it for the weekend? The bottom line is do not let intermittent fasting stop you from eating what you enjoy. Eat whatever you want, but always in moderation. Remember, the point here is to navigate the health world with positivity and happiness and denying yourself what you love will not result in contentment. In my opinion, the 16/8 fasting schedule is the best intermittent fasting choice you can make. By simply approaching it with the right attitude and working around your own emotions and preferences can go a long way in determining how successful your fasting experience can be.

Chapter 5: 16/8 For Women

Intermittent fasting is for one and all. Anyone willing to lose weight and live a healthy life is right for intermittent fasting. It is well suited for women who want to shed those extra pounds and reach fitness goals because a woman's health and body go through hills and valleys as they age. Right from the time a girl reaches maturity, marriage pregnancy, childbirth, breastfeeding and weaning, a woman's body undergoes a myriad of changes. And a woman with multiple children has experienced this change and shift many times, requiring specific work to see any improvement. It is a huge testament to the wonder of nature witnessing what a woman's body and mind can do.

In all this, if a lady wishes to lose weight, get her body back in shape and generally remain in good health, then there can be no better way to succeed than by following an intermittent fasting pattern, especially on the 16/8 schedule. The flexibility alone makes it a perfect fit by easily accommodating the challenges of a woman's rigorous home and work life.

Most experts agree that intermittent fasting with a fasting window of more than 24 hours is not advisable for most women. A fasting period of twelve to a maximum of sixteen hours is seen as the best option for a woman. This is because a woman's body is governed by several hormones that are interconnected in an extremely intricate way. A slight imbalance in one hormone can trigger a possible domino effect and cause other hormone productions to suffer also.

When a woman goes on a long fast, the body anticipates the oncoming famine and goes into self protection mode. Naturally, your body does not understand that you are voluntarily participating in a non-eating period, instead it only notices that food isn't coming in like it does normally and it seems as if no food will enter the body anytime soon either. Famine is obviously different from a self-imposed fast, but your body doesn't know that. To protect itself it shuts down all processes that could otherwise support another life within your body.

This is why even if a woman is not pregnant or trying to conceive, their body can still change, stop or disrupt the menstrual cycle so they are less likely to conceive while doing fasting. Not saying that you can't get pregnant during this time so it is best to always be safe, using normal contraception but it is a self preservation technique that the body can adopt to protect itself from continued lack of food and conserve resources.

So how can women fast so their bodies do not go into hormonal lockdown and remain at an optimal level? Is it safe for women and do they risk their very core of femininity by fasting intermittently? The answer to that question is yes, intermittent fasting is safe for women and there is a method to do it safely.

How Women Should Implement Intermittent Fasting

There are a few things that can be termed as drawbacks or disadvantages to intermittent fasting, such as dizziness, lightheadedness, nausea, extreme hunger, dehydration and so on. But all these are more or less similar for both men and women. Also, these mostly appear in the initial stages of intermittent fasting when the body is still getting used to going without food and beverages for a fixed number of hours. Once the body gets accustomed to the fasting hours, the fast will not seem so rigorous and things will get easier.

But, what can be bothersome is the disturbance to a woman's hormone levels and the irregularity of their menstrual cycles. This is what needs to be addressed first and foremost. There are a few steps that women can take to ensure their hormone levels are not disturbed and their desired weight loss goals are also achieved. Let's look at what these important measures can be.

Start Slow

This is extremely essential. You do not want your body to go into panic mode and take drastic measures when you suddenly begin fasting for longer hours. Start slowly with a 12 hour fast and build your 16 hour fast from there. Do not fast for more than 16 hours at a time. Also, make it a point to fast non-consecutive days. In the initial days, you can even restrict your fasts to two days a week. Do not fast for more than four days in a week and that too not on consecutive days. The aim here is to continuously give your body the assurance that you are not going hungry and you have meals at your disposal, at least every other day.

Hydration

If you are not taking in solids, then you need to give your body sufficient fluids to feel adequately hydrated. Drink plenty of non-caloric or low-calorie drinks like bone broth, plain black coffee, plain water, etc. You can even drink herbal tea in the initial days to let your body settle into the fasting schedule.

Eat Well

Make it a point to eat well in your eating window. Include green smoothies, fruits, and sufficient proteins in your meal. Take any supplements you might need to keep your vitamins and mineral levels consistent. Eating well in this window will reassure your body that you are not starving and have food at your disposal. If you eat restrictedly in your eating window it will send the wrong signals to your body. It will reaffirm your body's understanding of the situation that it is indeed starving or experiencing a lack of food. Remember, you do not want to eat junk, rather eat a whole and hearty meal, that leaves you feeling full and satisfied.

Placement of Your Eating Window

Where you have your eating window concerning your day and your regular activities determines how effective your fast is going to be. Women are naturally more susceptible and sensitive to a lack of food and the side effects. So, it's better to place your eating window to overlap with your most active hours so you will save your body from being burnt out. If your most active hours are afternoon to early evening, then place your eating window in those hours. Let your body accumulate sufficient energy through whole foods and when you are relaxed and not straining yourself physically, you can let your body experience the fast. It isn't to say that you mustn't do any physical work in the fasting state, take it slowly while engaging in light cardio, simple stretches, or walking.

Signs to Watch

Intermittent fasting can be highly beneficial to anyone who practices it. But when not done correctly, especially for women, intermittent fasting can pose some serious problems. Fortunately, there are few signs and signals that women can identify and take measures accordingly to counter the negatives of intermittent fasting. If these are just your initial stages, and first few days, they are not serious and your body's way of adjusting to the new schedule. If signals are persistent after two or three weeks you might want to consider changing your approach or even entirely reconsider going through with it.

Lack of Sleep

If you are experiencing a lack of sleep it might be a sign that your current intermittent fasting plan is not exactly working for you. Lack of sleep could be due to numerous reasons. Insufficient meals, hormonal changes, stress can all be reasons for lacking sleep. Your sleep time is your body's down time. It is the time your body uses to repair and correct any tissue injuries or cell breakage. While the first part of your sleep hours are used to correct physical injuries and repair your body, the latter half is used to resolve psychological issues like stress or anxiety you might be experiencing. This is primarily why we find ourselves awake in the middle of the night because our body is in a way urging us to address our problems and solve them. A fasting diet can result in considerable amounts of stress which can cause sleepless nights.

Lack of Focus

For some, a fasting diet can make it difficult to focus. Be it at work, or regular chores around the house, one might experience a lack of concentration or even interest in work when intermittent fasting is not done right, and it begins to influence the mind negatively. Intermittent fasting, when done correctly, is supposed to make you more alert and sharpen your focus, when this doesn't happen and instead you begin to notice the reverse of it, it might be a sign that your particular plan of fasting schedules isn't working correctly. You might need to tweak your plan a little and experiment around with it until you feel comfortable with what you have got.

Hair Loss

Hair loss is another sign that your fasting plan is adversely affecting your body. Many women undergo hormonal changes or depleted calories which can result in hair loss. For women especially, hair loss is one of the first signs that tell them their hormones are out of balance. You might want to change your fasting plans and see if it makes a difference or you might want to take a break from fasting for a while. Do consult your doctor if the problem persists.

Depression

Women might experience depression, anti-social behavior, and have higher anxiety levels while fasting as it is a common problem with anyone during this process. But, it is mostly present only in the first few days and then the heavy feelings disappear. Only when these feelings persist beyond this time and do not dissipate after a few weeks, then there might be a cause for concern. Depression can be the result of hormonal changes. Changing the intermittent fasting plan a little and reducing your fasting hours might help here. But if the problem persists, you might want to reconsider your decision to continue with any kind of fasting plan.

Orthorexia

This is a rare condition in people who fast intermittently. Orthorexia is an increased obsessiveness with one's food choices. This could be when you see yourself obsessing or worrying about your next meal, and the correctness of your choice of food, etc. Usually, this is seen with people who frequently practice and change their diets for weight loss. Diets induce a sense of oversensitivity in people. This occurs when the diet you are on is inflexible. This is why such obsessive worrying is less likely to occur with intermittent fasting because it can be managed and altered to fit any schedule. When you feel your intermittent fasting plan is rigid, with no scope for improvements or changes, it might be time to think over your plan and design a new strategy that helps manage anxiety.

Constant Irritation

This is another mild sign that you might need to tweak your fasting plan or change your approach. If you are constantly in an irritable mood, are usually angry and frustrated, then you might perhaps need to change your hours of fasting. Constant irritation will affect not just you but also the people in your family and all those around you, so if you feel yourself experiencing such constant irritation, take measures to change your plan. Taking a break from fasting or spacing out your fasts can also help curb such feelings.

Missed Periods

This is the most commonly observed sign amongst women. This is a solid indication that your hormonal balance has been disturbed. As discussed earlier, this occurs as your body's protection tactic. Women can experience irregular periods, complete lack of the menstrual cycle, or even shrunken ovaries. This occurs when your fasts are intense and last for longer durations. If you are fasting alternate fasts of 24-hours, and keep at it for months together, then you might experience irregular periods. This is why keep your fasts short, of only 14 to 16 hours, and space them out as two or three times a week.

Women who are pregnant, breastfeeding, or looking to conceive must not fast, even intermittently. Also, those women who have an eating disorder or are underweight must stay away from all forms of intermittent fasting.

Women who are nearing menopause or undergoing menopause might also experience additional stress. During this time women experience flashes of heat, palpitations, and irregular periods. Adding the stress of fasting can be difficult for a woman in this age group. For postmenopausal women, issues can arise after they have crossed this menopausal stage such as diabetes, unnatural weight gain, heart issues, etc. They do not have the risk of messing up their hormones very much as they are past the childbearing age. This is why intermittent fasting is the ideal way to lose weight and retain good health.

There are numerous instances where women were able to successfully participate in a 16/8 intermittent fast. They even achieved great results in losing their desired number of pounds and maintaining a healthy lifestyle. The key here is to let your body adapt to intermittent fasting slowly and sticking to basics of a 16/8 fast and not stretching yourself too much.

Chapter 6: Results From an 8-Week Study of 16/8 Fasting Experience

A study was conducted on 34 healthy individuals who were given a 16/8 intermittent fasting plan for over eight weeks. Seventeen individuals were given the time-restricted feeding plan while the remaining seventeen were allotted a normal diet.

Method

The time restricted feeding or TRF group was allowed to eat three meals in an eight-hour window. Three times were allotted to them at 1 pm, 4 pm, and 8 pm. The remaining hours from 8 pm to 1 pm the following day were the allotted fasting hours. For the normal diet group or ND group, three meal times were specified as breakfast at 8 am, lunch at 1 pm, and dinner at 8 pm. No meals or snacks were allowed for either group of participants in between meals. All the 34 participants were previously resistance-trained and continued a similar training pattern during the study.

All the groups were given a margin of one hour to complete their meals. Their caloric intake was standardized with a give and take of around 400 to 500 calories. The TRF group was given a standard caloric meal of around 2800 calories, give or take 500. Whereas the ND group was given a standard caloric meal of around 3100 calories. There wasn't much of a difference between the calories as the main focus was on the timing of the meal.

The two groups were also given standardized resistance training procedures to follow that were similar for both the groups. Training routines were divided into multiple sessions that each group had to follow. The routines were commonly followed and included the bicep curl, bench press, leg press, leg curl, leg extension, military press, incline dumbbell fly, wide and reverse grip pulldown, and tricep press. Being previously trained in resistance exercises the group was well acquainted with these exercises and felt no additional strain where someone new to training would have felt. This was tailored to produce results exclusive to the fasting schedules. The food calories were divided into varying percentages for breakfast, lunch, and dinner, or the three allotted meals for the fasting group. For the TRF group, the calorie percentages were divided as 40%, 25%, and 35% for their three respective meals. For the ND group, the calorie percentages were divided as 25%, 40%, and 35% for their three respective meals. The specific caloric percentages eaten by each group were assigned by a nutritionist and took into consideration the study subjects' inputs of their regular calorie intake.

The following are some of the results of this study. The study took into account muscle strength, fat loss, various hormone levels and so on.

Fat Mass

After the designated eight weeks, the body fat of both the groups was measured. The fat mass measurement was carried out using dual-energy Xray absorptiometry. The regular weights and heights of both the groups were measured using an electronic scale and a wall-mounted scale respectively. With respect to fat mass, the TRF group reported a considerable decrease while the ND group's fat mass remained more or less unchanged.

Lean Mass

Lean mass, muscle mass, or fat-free mass are all related as it is the measurement of muscle development in the body. For both groups, muscle mass was measured using an anthropometric tape at various sites in the body. Measuring the mid-arm, mid-thigh, biceps, triceps, and thighs were taken as the standards for this research to note any change in muscle mass or fat-free mass. Care was taken to ensure all the measurements were rounded off to the nearest 0.001m and were carried out by the same anthropometric tape and research official to confirm and establish stability and consistency in measurements. Here again, the

TRF group showed a remarkable improvement in lean mass, with an increased fat-free mass on the body, while the ND group remained more or less unchanged.

Muscle Strength

This was again a standard measurement for both the groups wherein subjects were tested for muscle strength during their resistance training sessions. During each session, the training was made slightly harder to test the strength of the subject's muscles. These were notably the same kind of sessions that the subjects could easily perform with a slightly lowered weight or load mass. For example, during a bench press session, the load was increased gradually until the subject could lift no more. The same was carried out with all the subjects for both the groups. The same training test was routinely carried out at varying intervals of time. Here again, the TRF group performed remarkably well. They showed great improvements in muscle strength and were able to lift and move weights that they would not have normally been able to. This was a clear testament to the fact that the 16/8 intermittent fasting schedule was indeed great at improving your muscle strength. The ND group's performance remained unchanged during the eight weeks.

Basal Metabolism

The basal metabolism rate for both the groups was measured intermittently for the whole eight week period. There was no particular change observed in either of the groups. The TRF group which was on the 16/8 fasting plan was assumed to have a lower rate of metabolism at the end of the study, but surprisingly the metabolic rate remained the same. This proved that intermittent fasting does not slow down the basal metabolic rate of the body as is commonly believed. The aggregate of both the groups' metabolic rates more or less remained the same.

Hormone Levels

Different hormones showed different results when measured for levels of presence in participants of both the groups. For example, the testosterone hormone remained unchanged for the ND group while the same was slightly reduced for the participants of the TRF group. This was measured with the aggregate of both total and free testosterone levels. Another hormone, insulin-like growth factor - 1 was also measured in both the groups and again was found unchanged in the ND group while it was slightly reduced in the TRF group. Hormones like leptin were also found with slightly decreased levels in the TRF group while they remain largely unchanged in the ND group. The thyroid hormones of T3, T4, and TSH were also measured. The TRF group showed a slight decrease in the T3 levels while showing no change in the thyroid stimulating hormone (TSH). Insulin was found to be remarkably lowered in fasting individuals of the TRF group, while for the ND group the insulin levels largely underwent several spikes throughout a day, all through the study.

Adiponectin, which is a proteinaceous hormone was seen to increase in the fasting individuals of the TRF group while it remained unchanged for the ND individuals.

Changes Observed in Biomarkers

Several biomarkers of health were monitored over the course of eight weeks that indicated the overall health of the participants of both the groups. The various biomarkers recorded were different lipid forms, blood glucose levels, cholesterol, heart disease risk factors, and so on. For the various lipid forms, the two groups remained more or less unchanged whereas triglycerides were significantly reduced in the TRF group. This again is a proof that the intermittent fasting schedules help cut down on the fat mass of your body. Triglycerides are the main kind of fat molecules that are widely present in an obese individual. The low levels of TG fats in a fasting individual proves that these can be significantly reduced using diligent eating times.

The ND group showed no change at all in the lipid levels of all kinds. The lipids measured mainly consisted of HDL, LDL, TRiglycerides, and total cholesterol. These are also considered as significant markers for the risk of heart disease, and other cardiovascular issues.

Respiratory Exchange Ratio

The respiratory exchange ratio of any organism or cell is the ratio of carbon dioxide that the said organism or cell produces during various processes like metabolism and the oxygen used to carry out the process. The lower the respiratory ratio the healthier and leaner a person is considered to be. These measurements are also known as the ventilatory measurements carried out using the fixed open circuit calorimetry. For each participant, the oxygen uptake and the carbon dioxide expelled were recorded breath by breath. The calorimeter was calibrated to the normal reference level of gases prior to testing each participant. The gas levels, both intake and expelled, were used to calculate the resting energy expenditure along with the respiratory exchange ratio for each participant using the modified Weir equation.

A significant decrease in the respiratory ratio was observed for the TRF group while the ND group's values remained unchanged. The respiratory ratio is high when an organism or cell is using a lot of carbon dioxide and is not making good use of oxygen. Low respiratory ratios mean oxygen is being put to good use through oxidation of lipids and other fats. This is a significant marker to prove the oxidation or breakdown of fats that occurs on account of a fasting schedule as seen in this study.

At the end of the study, the TRG group showed great differences through decreased overall fat mass, lean muscle growth, increased muscle strength, and reduced respiratory ratio. Slight changes were observed in the reduction of a few hormone levels like growth factor 1, testosterone, and T3. Encouraging changes were also observed in reduced leptin, insulin, and increased adiponectin levels. Various biomarkers were also observed to significantly reduce, indicating an improvement in health and a lower risk of disease.

It can be concluded that intermittent fasting is a great technique to help you lose weight and increase your lean muscle mass. According to this study, such a time-restricted feeding or the 16/8 schedule is ideal for athletes who need more lean muscle and decreased fat mass ratio. It is also well suited for otherwise healthy individuals who wish to lose weight and maintain good health.

Chapter 7: The Fat Loss Equation

Intermittent fasting is not a diet. We have established that. Intermittent fasting is a tool that you can use alone or along with any diet. Picking the right diet with the correct combination of macronutrients and coupling it with an intermittent fasting schedule, is a recipe for success in your weight loss program.

A calorie is a unit of energy that a body uses or consumes. For most people, calories indicate how food impacts their weight goals. For effective weight loss, most people stick to achieving a balance of calories consumed vs. calories burned. If one wishes to lose weight, they likely aim to consume a limited amount of calories while burning more than they consume. If one wishes to gain weight, then they do the opposite by consuming a higher number of calories than what is burned in exercise. For those who wish to manage their current size, a constant number of calories is maintained.

The biggest flaw here is treating all calories the same. No thought is given to the different nutrients that contribute to calorie count. Naturally, calories from a pound of fish is not the same as calories from a bowl of oats. Care must be given to what nutrients contribute to the total caloric count and what percentage is needed for effective weight loss. But before we begin to understand the role calories play, we need to get acquainted with the whole macronutrient phenomenon which makes the maximum contribution to calories we consume.

Understanding Macros

Having a thorough understanding of our macronutrients will help us in making the right decisions about our food. The three nutrients that are termed as the major contributors to our health are proteins, carbohydrates, and fats. The following three categories are known as the macronutrients or macros.

Protein

Proteins are essential components of all cells in the body. They are needed for good muscle growth. The most common sources of proteins are fish, chicken, meat, milk, eggs, and vegetables like beans and legumes.

Carbohydrates

These are the main energy providers. They are essential for various functions that are performed within our bodies at the cell level. They are also required for any and every function we do. The most common sources of carbs are sugars and starch products like wheat, rice, various grains, sugars, potatoes, and other starchy vegetables.

Fats

Most people believe that fats are bad. According to many, the more fats they shed the better it is, and this is why people avoid eating fats in any form. But fats are essential components of our diet. We need fat because they help us keep warm and protect our organs. They are also necessary for cell growth and lend a hand in the absorption of some nutrients. Various dry fruits and nuts, oils, butter or cream, and a few types of fish are great sources of fats.

Most diets treat food and calories under the one size fits all phenomenon. This is not always true, nor is it helpful to what your body really needs. Each individual is different and has different needs. What might work for one individual with one kind of needs and goal in mind might not work for another who has an entirely different goal in mind and has different needs.

Understanding where the calories are coming from, what macros are and what percentage of each macro we need in our diet can help us make more informed choices.

People often measure their weight loss success or failure in terms of their numbers on the scale. It is the scale that rules. Weight loss cannot be equal to losing fat. Sure, your scale shows you lost a couple of pounds in the last month with the help of your rigorous diet, but are you sure that the weight loss is from fat reduction and not water loss, muscle loss, or something else entirely? Scales cannot tell the difference. So how can we be sure that what we are losing is indeed fat?

There are a few methods in place that can help you calculate what amount of each nutrient you will need to help lose fat. This can seem long and drawn out with so much math involved, but taking it one step at a time will help you reach there. Before you begin your calculations, take a deep breath, calm yourselves and give this your attention. It might look intimidating, but it is the simplest of ways to ensure your diets are true and effective.

10 Step Macro Calculation

For calculating your macronutrient requirements, we need to follow a few simple rules. There are ten basic steps that can lead you to your correct combination of macros.

Calculate BMR

The first step is to calculate your BMR. BMR is the measure of your basal metabolic rate. It is the energy units that your body spends when at rest. Energy is required for various functions within our body and BMR helps you determine the number of energy units one needs. There are various ways you can calculate your BMR, through equations, through BMR calculators, or through diet and nutrition professionals.

Below is a simple equation that can give you your BMR values in a simple way.

Mifflin-St Jeor Equation

This equation gives two separate formulas for men and women based on their height, weight, age, etc. You will simply need to substitute your specs into the equation, run the simple math, and you will have your BMR.

Women:

BMR = 10 x weight (kg) + 6.25 x height (cm) - 5 x Age (yrs) - 161

Men:

BMR = 10 x weight (kg) + 6.25 x height (cm) - 5 x Age (yrs) + 5

Activity Level

While BMR gives you energy expended while at rest, activity level value or activity factor is a measure of a person's level of activeness. Different people are comfortable at different levels of activity in their lives. Some are more sedentary, while others are super active and athletic. Both these groups naturally cannot have the same caloric requirement and will need different macros percentages for effective weight loss. Mostly the activity levels are divided into six different categories as sedentary, lightly active, moderately active, active, very active and athletic.

Sedentary - You are not active at all or are injured and cannot do any form of exercise. The activity factor is 1.2.

Lightly active - You are minutely active. You might not work out as much, but go for an occasional walk, or enjoy light work around the house. The activity factor is 1.3.

Moderately active - You do house chores, or light cardio, walk or run regularly. The activity factor is 1.4.

Active - You make it a point to stay active, you workout at least five times a week. The activity factor is 1.55.

Very active - You are on your toes. You have a demanding day job or you are required to stand for more than five hours a day. The activity factor is 1.7

Athletic - You are extremely active. You work out for at least three hours every day. The activity factor is 1.9.

Total Daily Energy Expenditure

Total daily energy expenditure is the measure of how much energy you spend on a daily basis. This is the number of calories that you need to maintain your current body mass after you have accounted for the calories that you require for your current body weight at rest, which is the BMR, and the calories for your particular activity level, which is the activity factor.

TDEE = BMR calculated above x Activity Factor.

Establish Your Weight Goal

This is where you find out what exact number of calories you will need to achieve your weight goal. Your goal could be anything, from weight loss through fat burn, or weight maintenance, or even gaining lean muscle mass.

The TDEE values are used as a base for calculating your goal. This gives you the number of calories you should ideally consume to reach your goal.

If you wish to burn one pound of body fat per week, then you are required to burn at least 3500 calories in the seven days. This would amount to 500 calories per day. So, using this standard to calculate your weight goal, you will have:

Fat Loss

For losing fat we will need to subtract 500 calories from the TDEE per day values.

Fat loss calories = TDEE - 500

Weight Maintenance

For maintaining your weight, you will need the same TDEE values to be maintained.

Maintenance calories = TDEE

Muscle Gain

For muscle gain, you need to add 500 calories to the TDEE values as the reverse of the fat-loss equation.

Muscle gain calories = TDEE + 500

Through our goal determining process, we have identified the number of calories we will need to burn fat, maintain our weight or gain muscle. Now is the time to individually identify what each macronutrient's contribution will be to the total calories.

Identify Macros

To determine macronutrient percentage in calories we need to decide on the reasons for our set weight loss goal. There are various methods to work out your macros but here we shall concentrate on two main approaches that are widely practiced around the world.

The 'Regular' Approach

This is also known as the more mainstream way. Here you need a low fat plan. The carbs and proteins are equally distributed in a meal. The basic percentages of the different macros in this approach are as follows:

Proteins: 35% to 40%

Carbs: 35% to 45%

Fats: 15% to 30%

The mainstream approach is ideal for those with a time restriction and no major health issues. This is great for anyone looking to lose less than or equal to 20% of their current body weight. Models and actors mostly follow this approach. Any individual with a timed fat loss goal or want a muscular, lean appearance, this approach is ideal for you.

The Keto Approach

This is popular among those with diabetes and other ailments. Individuals who are insulin resistant, have PCOS, or are undergoing hormonal shifts such as perimenopausal women in the stages before menopause are best suited for this approach. People who have difficulty digesting, processing and absorbing starches, or need to lose more than 50 pounds, this is best for you. The basic percentages of the various macros in this approach are as follows:

Proteins: 20% to 25%

Carbs: 5%

Fats: 70% to 75%

This is an extremely low carb and high fat plan that helps you navigate carb issues and insulin problems that one might have.

Based on what your weight goals are and for what purpose and your body needs, you can decide what approach will suit your weight loss regimen. You can then plan specific macro contributions for your own caloric needs. This will help you reach the ideal macro percentage that can give you a sustainable weight loss program. combining this with your intermittent fasting schedule will only make your weight loss aim that much surer to achieve.

Protein Consumption

Determine your protein consumption from the standard requirements for an individual based on a person's activity level. For example, an individual with a sedentary lifestyle and no workout regime, the recommended protein intake is 0.4 to 0.6g per pound of body mass. Similarly, for people who are lightly active, the recommended protein intake is 0.7 to 0.8g per pound of body mass. For those who are active, the intake is around 0.8 to 1g per pound of body mass and extremely active individuals, thei intake is 1 to 1.5g per pound of body mass.

You can also follow the FDA guidelines which recommend 10% of the total consumed calories to come from proteins or the World Health Organization (WHO) guidelines direct protein consumption of an individual be at 0.8g per kg.

Fat Consumption

The FDA and WHO recommend a total of 30% of calories to come from fats for general good health when there are no adverse health indicators to this proposition.

For people wishing for moderate fat loss, the recommended fat intake is 0.30g to 0.40g per pound of body mass. For those following the keto diet, the desired fat intake is 70 to 75% of total calories.

Carbohydrate Consumption

According to the FDA and WHO the recommended carb intake must be 300 to 400 grams per day. For keto dieters, the desired carb consumption is a low percentage of only 5% of the total calories. For fat loss purposes the carb intake is set at 0.7 to 1.5g per pound of body mass. 1.5 to 2g per pound of body mass is taken as a standard for those who wish to maintain their current body weight.

Now that we have established the intake in grams of the three different macronutrients, let's now move onto calculating the whole fat loss equation with respect to these macros. With our determined macro intake, we can find the number of calories our body needs and the percentage of macronutrient contribution in those calories that are specific to us.

Macronutrient Fat Loss Template

We begin by calculating the daily calorie goal for our bodies when we are aiming at efficient fat loss. You can do similar equations for maintenance and muscle growth goals too.

- BMR x Activity Factor = TDEE

TDEE - 500 = Daily calorie goal for fat loss

- Grams of protein/lb x goal weight = Total protein

Total protein x 4 cal/ gram of protein = Calories from proteins

- Grams of fat/lb x goal weight = Total fats

Total fat x 9 cal/gram of fat = Calories from fats

- Daily calorie goal - (calories from proteins + calories from fats) = Calories from carbs cal from carbs ÷ 4 cal/gram of carbs = Grams of carbs

Now that we have the grams of all three macronutrients and their caloric contribution, we can easily determine the percentage of their contributions as follows:

- Daily calorie goal ÷ cal from proteins = % of proteins
- Daily calorie goal ÷ cal from proteins = % of fats
- Daily calorie goal ÷ cal from carbs = % of carbs

Review and Final Macro Count

This is the last and final step where you review your macro numbers and its effect on your health and lifestyle. You would most likely combine the above-achieved numbers of macro percentages into your eating habits around intermittent fasting schedules. You would need to review the way your body is reacting to your assigned food percentages.

Consider whether the carbs you are consuming will give you enough satisfaction and a feeling of fullness. Will the carbs be enough to fuel your workouts and other activities? Is the high protein content too overwhelming if you are not used to it? Are the calories sufficient and going at a rate that is suitable for you? Is the food too much to include in your eating windows? So and so forth, you can review your macro number from all angles. You could even tweak them a little to suit your preferences better, but do not deteriorate much from the path, because in the end, the number suggests what suits your goals and lifestyle best.

This fat loss macronutrient template only gives you a guideline to follow when you aim for a moderate fat loss regime. Using the same technique as above you can determine your numbers for maintenance of your body weight and also for gaining lean muscle mass. You will simply have to substitute the variables with your numbers and calculate using the equations. This is a great way to ensure your calories are the perfect combination and was designed so that it can have the maximum impact on your weight goals.

As an example, take an individual, a female with a moderately active lifestyle looking for fat loss. Let's calculate the macro percentages for this individual. The person weighs 74 kilos, with a goal weight of 62 kilos. The BMR for this individual is 1469. As the person is moderately active the activity factor would be 1.4.

The TDEE would then be, 1390 x 1.4 = 2056

Fat loss caloric goal or daily calorie goal would be, 1946 - 500 = 1556

As the person is moderately active, the protein intake would be 122g

Calories from protein would be 122 x 4 = 488

The fat intake for this person would be 40.8g

Calories from fats would be 40.8 x 9 = 367

Calories from carbs = Daily calorie goal - (protein cal + fat cal) = 1556 - (488 + 367) = 701 = calories from carbs.

Carb intake is Calories from carbs ÷ 4 = 701 ÷ 4 = 175g

So now the caloric percentages of each macro would be as follows:

Percentage of protein = Cal from protein ÷ daily calorie goal = 488 ÷ 1556 x 100 = 32%

Percentage of Fats = Cal from fats ÷ daily calorie goal = 367 ÷ 1556 x 100 = 23%

Percentage of Carbs = Cal from carbs ÷ daily calorie goal = 701 ÷ 1556 x 100 = 45%

The person would be required to take their daily calories according to the below percentages:

- Protein - 32%
- Fats - 23%
- Carbs - 45%

Many people equate this to fad diets that are in style or trending, but in reality, this is not true. The fat loss equations we have seen above give you the freedom of adjusting your macro intake based on your lifestyle, your activity level, your biological buildup, and your ultimate weight goal. All these particulars are absent in the fad diets that stick to a fixed number of calories.

In the end, when you are satisfied with what numbers you have come up with, make it a point to place a chart or some such pointer at a visible place to keep yourself motivated and firm on the path of fat loss. Here you can enter these numbers and your preferences in your journal. This will help you compare what number or percentages of macros had you feeling well and confident and what numbers left you wanting and hungry. Weave this into your intermittent fasting schedules for optimum results.

Chapter 8: Metabolism

Your metabolism is the process your body uses to convert food into energy. Here the calories produced from food are combined with oxygen to generate energy. The rate at which this process takes place is known as the metabolic rate. The basal metabolic rate is the number of calories required by the body to perform its normal bodily functions when at rest. Many people believe that fasting decreases the metabolic rate of your body. When a person goes without food for really longer durations, it causes a drop in the body's metabolism. But is this true for intermittent fasting too?

During an intermittent fast, and especially the 16/8 intermittent fasting protocol which is our subject of study here, it is an entirely different case.

Our metabolic rate indeed increases when eaten food is being converted into energy but that is not the only method by which our bodies have a healthy metabolic rate. There are many different factors and processes that affect the metabolic rate of our body. Intermittent fasting might restrict the food intake for sure, but it definitely enhances the other factors and processes that increase or maintain our metabolic rate. It is important to understand that the thermic effect of food is not the only source of metabolic spike that a person might experience.

Thermic Effect of Food

It is the rate of energy expenditure that our body uses to digest, absorb, and store food. This is in addition to the basal metabolic rate which is calculated at rest. Some foods require larger quantities of energy for our bodies to be able to digest, assimilate, and store the resulting nutrients. These foods are known as high thermic effect foods. They result in large spikes in your metabolic rate when you eat them and might be a good way to keep your metabolism running at a high level. Naturally, it only lasts as long as food digestion and assimilation occurs. Such high thermic effect foods are protein-rich foods like eggs, fish, meat, dairy products, nuts, etc. Also, it is essential to note that metabolic rate falls when there are fewer calories consumed. Intermittent fasting, in general, does not restrict calorie consumption as much as it does the time of the food consumed. One can continue a diet of 2000 calories with ease while still ˋpracticing intermittent fasting.

Factors Stabilizing Metabolic Rate While Intermittent Fasting

Now let's look at the different factors that ensure your metabolic rate does not drop while intermittent fasting.

Increase in Human Growth Hormone (HGH)

This is one of the biggest advantages of intermittent fasting. Intermittent fasting helps increase the levels of human growth hormone or HGH in the bloodstream. HGH is an essential hormone that promotes muscle growth and the oxidation of fats. This alone ensures that the metabolic processes within your body do not stop and continue at a stable rate. The 16/8 fast, in particular, is ideal for not letting your metabolic rate drop.

It has also been observed by intermittent fasting practitioners that a week of intermittent fasting schedules increases your HGH levels by over 1200%! That is an amazing level of HGH hormone to aim for and it sure keeps your metabolic processes running.

Drop in Insulin Levels

We have seen earlier how insulin packs our sugars into fat and stores them for later. It is therefore understandable that it is close to impossible for our bodies to break down fats when the insulin levels are high. It is a fat-storing hormone and would naturally not allow for the fat to be broken down. Now, any oxidative process resulting in energy can be termed metabolism. For this very exact reason, during intermittent fasting, as the insulin levels drop, our body begins to move onto fats to burn or oxidize to produce energy. This is how a drop in insulin levels keeps the metabolic process of fat oxidation going.

Increase in Norepinephrine Hormone Levels

Norepinephrine is a stress hormone released by our body. It is the flight or fight hormone that is released when the body senses itself in a difficult or dire situation. Here high levels of norepinephrine hormone mean an increased breakdown of fats. Seeing it like this, when the body senses it is in a restricted food phase it increases the norepinephrine levels, which in turn direct it to the stored fat to meet energy needs. Seeing as the 16/8 fast is short and not very intense in its implementation, this increase in stress hormone is short-lived. While it lasts, it directs the body to burn fat and because it doesn't stay so for long it doesn't bring about any new adverse influences on the body.

Active Muscle Tissue

Muscle cells and muscle tissue are constantly undergoing active metabolic processes of their own. Digestion of food alone is not the only metabolic process in our body. Whenever energy is produced by oxidation of nutrients it is called metabolism. For example, during an exercise regimen, the muscles can account for the consumption of over 60% of oxygen in our body. Muscles need the oxidative process to contract, which is their primary function. Also, anaerobically, or in other words in the absence of oxygen too, muscles are able to contract and perform their function for a time. This again is known as their metabolic processes and intermittent fasting promotes this muscle activity. First, you might be exercising, walking, or working while intermittent fasting. Second, intermittent fasting helps to keep muscles intact. Other fad diets or calorie-restricted dieting plans not just burn fats but also run the risk of burning muscle tissue. A dieter might not just lose fat but may also lose muscle. This is not the case with intermittent fasting. It helps you retain your muscle while burning just fat and, in some cases, also helps grow more lean muscle mass. This is a huge advantage of intermittent fasting.

In a study conducted on eleven healthy individuals who undertook the 16/8 fasting schedule, it was found in the end that their metabolic rates increased by about 14%. This is against what is commonly believed in relation to intermittent fasting and proves how intermittent fasting, when done right, cannot lower your metabolic rate. If it cannot increase, it will at least not let it drop. It is important to remember that it is the calories that spike or drop the metabolic rate. So, if a person is intermittent fasting, but eats very little during their eating window it can naturally result in a drop in metabolic rate.

For people with small appetites or those who restrict calories, eating limitedly will naturally cause the metabolic rate to drop whether they do intermittent fasting or not. And our metabolic rate spikes and drops from the time we begin eating to the time we finish our meal. So ideally, it is impossible to sustain a constant level of metabolic rate. We should instead aim at having fewer spikes and lows, and prevent it from falling too far short of the ideal for our body type. And intermittent fasting helps us do exactly that.

Chapter 9: Strategic Black Coffee

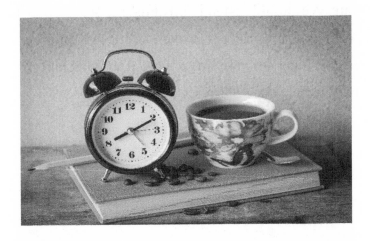

There are many theories out there supporting different kinds of beverages while intermittent fasting. But, black coffee is one that has the approval from all corners of the intermittent fasting world. Practitioners of intermittent fasting have been drinking straight black coffee, without milk or sugar, for as long as intermittent fasting has been around.

Benefits of Black Coffee

There are several amazing benefits of drinking black coffee sans the sugar, that make it a special drink for everyone whether fasting or not. Let's look at a few of those benefits that make coffee special.

Improves Cognition

Black coffee, when consumed regularly, has shown to improve a person's brain function. It works by increasing the dopamine levels and also has an activated psychoactive stimulant that works by improving the brain's focus and memory. Black coffee also helps keep various neurodegenerative disorders like Parkinson's, Alzheimer's, and dementia at bay. With increasing age, our cognitive abilities deteriorate, and we run a high risk of suffering from these diseases. Drinking black coffee every morning helps keep your brain active and also enhances the alertness of nerves. It is believed that drinking black coffee regularly can reduce the risk of Alzheimer's by 65% and that of Parkinson's by around 70%.

Aids in Weight Loss

Black coffee increases the adrenaline levels in the blood which readies your body for strenuous physical exercises. This is why it is always great to have a cup of black coffee before your workout as this can improve your physical performance. Adrenaline released in the bloodstream prepares for this physical exertion by burning fats into freely available fatty acids that are in turn used as fuel or energy for the physical exercise. Black coffee also enhances your metabolism by up to 50%. It is known as a fat-burning drink as it stimulates the brain into signaling the breakdown of fats.

Improves Liver Health

Black coffee is termed as a friend for the liver as it greatly improves liver health. It is known to keep liver diseases like cancer, hepatitis, fatty liver, and liver cirrhosis at bay. It has also been seen that people who drink at least four cups of black coffee have an 80% less chance of getting any kind of liver disease.

Diuretic

Coffee is a known diuretic which means it makes you urinate frequently. This is a great way to flush out toxins and other harmful substances from the body through urine. This helps to cleanse our bodies effectively. It is important to also stay hydrated with water.

Vitamins and Antioxidants

Black coffee has a horde of antioxidants and various vitamins such as B2, B3, and B5. It has a lot of other trace elements such as manganese, magnesium, and potassium which are essential micronutrients.

Reduces Risk of Diabetes and Cardiovascular Issues

Type 2 diabetes later gives rise to more serious problems like heart diseases and organ damage. Drinking coffee regularly helps reduce the risk of getting diabetes drastically. Drinking at least two cups of coffee daily greatly reduces the risk of cardiovascular diseases. It also reduces inflammation within the body and reduces the chances of a stroke.

Improves Mood

Stress and tension not only bring our moods down but can potentially bring about various serious health issues later on. Drinking black coffee helps fight depression. It stimulates the brain into releasing various neurotransmitters like serotonin, noradrenaline, etc., that help improve our mood drastically. Drinking a cup of coffee when we are feeling down and sad can make us feel better immediately.

Incorporating Black Coffee in an Intermittent Fasting Schedule

Black coffee can be a great choice while intermittent fasting. To glean maximum benefit from your cup of black coffee, make sure you follow these simple tips:

- Drink coffee only during your fasting hours and not during your eating window. Straight black coffee is a great way to blunt hunger.

- Do not have coffee first thing in the morning. Your cortisol levels are high in the morning, and having coffee will only lend it a further spike, which when it comes down can cause severe hunger.

- Wait for your cortisol levels to naturally come down, which it will after some time after you wake up in the morning. Drink a glass or two of plain cool water or sparkling water if you'd like.

- Have your first cup of coffee at least two to three hours after waking up.

- Divide your total coffee intake into two or more portions and space them out evenly throughout your fast.

- During a fast always take your coffee black and plain, without sugar.

- To have control over hunger, make it a point to sip your coffee slowly rather than drinking it all in one go.

- Opt for a dark roasted coffee blend if available because coffee has several compounds other than caffeine that can help fight hunger. And as dark roasted coffee has less caffeine it will not interfere with your sleep and also be beneficial to you at the same time.

Black coffee is an amazing choice of drink to include in your intermittent fasting schedule. If you are not used to drinking coffee or like your coffee with a bit of milk, cream, or sugar, you can work toward getting used to drinking straight black coffee. Implement the following simple tips to make your transition to sugarless milkless coffee easier.

- Gradually decrease your sugar intake. If you previously took a teaspoon of sugar with your cup of coffee, reduce about ⅕ teaspoon of sugar each day to completely wean yourself off sweet coffee.

- Try adding a pinch of salt into your cup of coffee to nullify the overpowering bitter taste.

- You can replace milk and sugar with other natural taste enhancers like cinnamon. Add a dash of cinnamon to your coffee either while you are brewing it or after it's brewed.

- You can also try adding a few drops of vanilla essence to your coffee to enhance its taste and counter the bitterness to some degree.

- In the initial days, take tiny sips of coffee and let your tongue really taste the flavor of the coffee beans. Coffee can be an acquired taste, and if you take the time to feel the flavor you can really get used to it.

- There are various blends and roasts available. If you find instant coffee suits you then it is perfectly fine, otherwise, you can buy your own coffee beans and grind them or buy ground coffee, while trying different roasts. Each roast is characterized by the color of the bean, and each has its own flavor. experiment with different blends to see what fits you best.

In the end, it is important to do what is good and right for your body, while keeping your own likes and preferences satisfied.

Chapter 10: Four Important Healthy Habits for Life

For any person to be healthy and sustain that good health there are four important things to take care of. These vital factors of good health are necessary for every individual despite gender or age. Let's look at what these four factors are that make up the healthy picture of our lives.

Nutrition

Eating good healthy whole foods is essential for our wellbeing. We hear it time and again that whole foods are best and the way to go to achieve good health. But what exactly are whole foods?

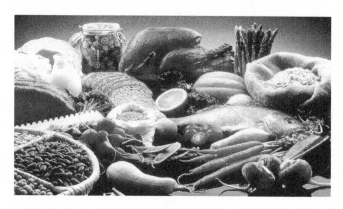

Whole Foods

Whole foods are single-ingredient foods that are 'whole' and relatively unprocessed. Foods such as fruits, vegetables, whole grains, nuts, seeds, or legumes come under the whole foods category. Unprocessed animal food can also be called as whole food.

All food is processed to some extent whether it be washing, cutting, chopping, boiling, canning, and so on. But foods that are as close to the state they were in when they were harvested are still termed as whole foods. The problems arise when further processing is done. As more and more processing techniques are employed in foods, they begin to lose their nutritive value. Processing such as adding various chemical additives, preservatives, taste boosters, and other chemical agents vastly diminishes the natural benefits a food has.

Nowadays, with the growing nutritional demands and preferences and the popularity of fad diets, people are forgetting the goodness that a wholesome meal provided. There are many advantages to be had by eating good whole foods. Whole foods are packed with nutrients while processed foods are simply energy-rich or calorie-rich foods.

- Whole foods have high amounts of fiber, minerals, and vitamins. Just one cup of peppers or orange slices is richer in vitamin C than a glass of processed orange juice.

- Whole foods are actually low in sugar. Indeed, fruits have sugar but they also have essential nutrients like vitamins and minerals along with fiber. Processed fruit juices, on the other hand, are loaded with added sugars, preservatives, and artificial colors.

- Whole foods are full of healthy fats that are good for your heart. Processed foods have 'bad' fats added like saturated or trans fats.

- The fiber content in whole foods is very high, which helps us with digestive processes and metabolism. It is this fiber that gives us the feeling of fullness and it is why we feel fuller when we eat whole foods when compared to eating processed foods that leave us feeling hungry.

- Whole foods help control our blood sugar and are good for keeping diabetes at bay.

- Whole foods also improve the health of our skin. They are full of antioxidants and vitamins that are good for our skin. Eating whole foods regularly helps combat issues like early wrinkles and loss of skin elasticity.

- Whole foods are great money savers. Processed foods while being unhealthy and downright harmful for our bodies can cost more than the organic alternative.

- Whole foods also help reduce unhealthy food cravings and overeating. As it contains fibers and keeps us full, it naturally diminishes cravings for sugars and foods like cakes, cookies, etc.

- Processed foods with their processed sugars and refined ingredients create dental cavities and decay. This is absent in whole foods which with their natural sugars actually improve our dental health.

- Whole foods are great at keeping diseases like cardiovascular issues, increased cholesterol, etc.
- Whole foods are also better for the environment because they do not include any nonbiodegradable material or processes that can harm nature. Apart from being nature friendly, consuming whole foods makes us farmer-friendly too.

How to Incorporate Whole Foods While Intermittent Fasting

During your eating window, make it a point to include whole foods like fruits, vegetables, whole, and unrefined grains, nuts, and legumes, etc. in your diet. Also include unprocessed meat products like fish, chicken, and egg. Avoid foods such as bacon, sausages, ham, and deli meats. For the most part of your fasting plan, try to eat as many whole foods as you can. Let around 80% of your fasting plan to comprise whole foods while you allow 20%

for your favorite comfort foods. If you are planning to fast for a week, eat whole foods for 80% of the week and your choice of food for the remaining 20%. Remember, the fewer the ingredients and the lesser the food is processed, the better it is for our health.

Sleep

Sleep is as essential to our body as food, water, and air. We hardly realize the importance of a good night's sleep. Sleeping the recommended seven to nine hours per night is necessary to keep our body functioning normally. Sleep is the time our body repairs itself and restores the body's various chemical balances. When we go sleepless, our body is unable to perform its function and no repairs and restorations take place. Signs of sleep deprivation include irritability, excess fatigue, repeated yawning, loss of focus, and loss of a sense of balance. Sleep deprivation is a serious problem and can result in a lot of problems for us both physically and emotionally.

Effects of Sleep Deprivation

Let's look at how sleep deprivation can harm the different system functions in our body.

The Nervous System

Sleep deprivation causes our brain to become sluggish and dull. The nervous system is the way our body sends and receives messages from within itself and also from around itself. But lack of sleep can make this whole transmission of messages faulty. Sleep is necessary to keep the system functioning properly. It is during sleep that connections are formed between neurons that help us remember what we have learned. Sleep also addresses any emotional stress we are going through. When this doesn't occur our brain begins to lose focus, and its retaining power diminishes. Lack of sleep can also make your responses and actions slower. It can make you more prone to accidents. Your creative faculties and decision-making abilities are also affected by lack of sleep.

Immune System

While we sleep, our body produces various agents that help us fight off infections and foreign invaders in our bodies like bacteria and viruses. During sleep, cytokines are produced by the body that strengthen our immune system and prepare our body against diseases. When there is a definite lack of sleep, we become more prone to diseases and also take longer to get better from illnesses and heal ourselves.

Digestive System

Along with the nervous system the biggest effect lack of sleep has is on our digestive system. One of the main reasons for weight gain and overeating is continued lack of sleep. Insufficient sleep messes up the hormones in our body that control the hunger and satiety signals. This is mostly why people feel excessive hunger at night and fall into the trap of unhealthy nighttime snacking. This is also the reason why our body produces more insulin when we eat than is normal which in turn causes increased fat storage and also increases the risk of type 2 diabetes.

Cardiovascular System

We need sleep to maintain a healthy heart. The entire cardiovascular system repairs itself during this downtime. When it is absent, we run a greater risk of injury and developing heart disease. One study even linked insomnia and continued lack of sleep to heart attacks.

Endocrine System

The effective, regular release of hormones is greatly dependent on sleep. Hormones such as Testosterone need a minimum of three hours of uninterrupted sleep to be released in the bloodstream.

Similarly, the growth hormones produced by the pituitary gland need sufficient sleep hours for effective release. These hormones are essential for muscle buildup and also repair of muscle cells and tissues. Especially in kids, lack of sleep can prove detrimental to growth as it hinders the release of these growth hormones.

How to Combat Sleep Deprivation

After being sleep deprived for such a long time, it's hard to find that normal sleep level again. But there are a few things that you can do to help yourself to sleep better:

- Avoid sleeping during the daytime. It can take away from your nighttime hours of sleep. Most people who nap in the day, fall asleep later during the night.

- Do not consume caffeine after lunch, or past noon. Caffeine consumption can greatly interfere with sleep time.

- Form a schedule and stick to it. Make it a point to sleep at the same time every night, and wake up at the same time every morning.

- Stick to your schedule every day, including weekends and holidays. At least until you are back to sleeping normally, you need to be firm with yourself.

- Prepare yourself mentally and physically for bed. Put on a pair of comfortable pajamas, play light music, burn a relaxing scent if you enjoy it. At least an hour before bed, make a point to do relaxing activities that don't involve screens such as reading, listening to music, meditating, or taking a bath.

- Finish your meals at least two hours before bedtime. You do not want your body to feel heavy and uncomfortable right before you hit the bed. In short, do not delay your dinner and eat early!

- Avoid using electronic devices like smartphones, TVs, computers, or tablets right before you go to bed.

- Include regular exercise in your schedule. Do not exercise right before bed but include some form of physical exercise in your daily schedule for the day.

- You can have a glass of warm milk as your last food an hour or so before sleeping.

If sleeping issues persist, it is better to consult a doctor and take professional advice to keep yourself healthy and sleeping well!

Exercise

The fact that exercise can keep you healthy is a well-known truth. Yet, very few people truly believe or follow this to be in good health. Let's first understand what exercise truly means. Exercise is any form of regular physical exertion that we push our bodies into. Activities like walking, running, jogging, swimming, etc. can all be termed as exercises. Exercises can also be weight training, resistance training, cardio exercises and so on. Exercising by whatever way we are comfortable with at least thrice a week can have huge benefits both mentally and physically.

Benefits of Exercise

- Exercise can help you build muscle. Exercise mainly concerns the skeletal system and doing them regularly will strengthen your muscles and bones.

- Exercise helps you with weight loss. Workouts of any kind push your body into burning fats and can be a great tool for weight loss.

- With exercise, you will be able to burn your glycogen stores quickly and move on to fat stores for energy and this is what will aid in weight loss.

- It has also been seen that exercise helps the release of hormones effectively.

- Exercises help with boosting your stamina and energy levels.

- Exercise speeds up your heart rate which pumps in more oxygenated blood to your brain. This can improve brain function and enhance memory skills.

- Exercising regularly can help you sleep better. Including some form of physical exercise in your daily schedule will ensure you sleep for longer continuous hours at night.

Supplements

Though supplements are not that necessary when you are intermittent fasting, it can become essential when you are on a keto diet or fasting for long durations of time. You will have to ensure you have enough levels of sodium, potassium, and magnesium. Make it a point to include health supplements that boost good health rather than exercise supplements that are meant for people doing long workouts and help in muscle building. Some supplements that you want to make sure your diet includes are vitamin D, magnesium, multivitamin, or fish oil supplements, etc. Always consult your doctor before including or combining any supplements with dieting or exercise.

Keeping all these four factors in good control will ensure you have a healthy mind and body. The absence of any one of these can greatly impact your health and is bound to invite diseases to your door.

Chapter 11: Intermittent Fasting FAQ and Facts

What's the best time for my fasting window?

Starting your fast as late at night as you can is the best way to maximize fat burn. Being active during the day while fasting will ensure you burn glycogen faster and move to fats earlier, so you have a longer fat-burning period. Starting your fast early on in the night will not help you as much as you are inactive and sleeping for most of the fast.

What can I do about bloating?

Bloating can be a problem especially in the early days of intermittent fasting. Possible causes of bloating can be hormonal changes, increased water intake, and so many other reasons. Especially if your body is not used to drinking a lot of water, it will initially hold on to it since it knows it doesn't normally get enough. If this is the reason, then there is nothing to worry about as it will sort itself out as you go along. Another reason for bloating could be any food intolerances you might have such as dairy, gluten, etc. You can sort through this by a trial and error method by taking out one food at a time and seeing if it makes a difference.

Will practicing fasting lead to binge eating?

Intermittent fasting need not necessarily lead to binge eating. But taking care to avoid a few common mistakes will help you overcome the urge to overeat. For example, break your fast with proper whole foods that keep you feeling fuller longer. Practice mindfulness to stay focused on your fast and keep motivated to stop yourself from breaking your fast or overeating. Start your intermittent fasting slowly and make it a point to eat well in your eating window.

Will stevia break my fast?

Stevia is not true sugar, but it is processed and has calories and will break your fast. But it depends on how serious you are taking your fasting. If your intention in practicing intermittent fasting is healing and body cleansing, you will have to stay away from it. But, if you simply want to lose some weight and want a way to do that without the fuss of meal prepping, eating six times a day, while also being able to enjoy bigger meals then stevia won't affect your fasts or stop you from achieving this.

Does fasting cause muscle loss?

No, as we have discussed earlier in the book, intermittent fasting promotes lean muscle growth and only burns fats.

Do calories matter when fasting

There is enough research out there that supports both theories that total calories do matter even with fasting as well as the fact that weight loss is purely hormonal. It can be your own individual understanding. I believe in most cases calories do matter at least to some extent and if you eat more than you burn off you won't lose weight even if you fast.

Can I apply any diet to intermittent fasting?

Yes, as discussed earlier, intermittent fasting is more a tool than an actual diet.

When is the best and worst time to train when following a 16/8 fasting schedule?

The worst time to exercise is the first few hours in the morning. Working out will cause hunger issues and since you have a few hours of fasting ahead of you it can make it more challenging. The best time to work out would be right before you are due to break your fast. And yet, if for some reason the only available time to you for workouts is early in the morning, then this is still better than not working out at all.

Who should not do 16/8 fasting?

Pregnant or breastfeeding women, women who are trying to get pregnant, people with type 1 diabetes, people with a history of eating disorders or are underweight, and individuals under 18 years of age.

People who are on prescribed medication, have gout or high uric acid, or people who have a history of or are currently suffering from liver, kidneys, or heart disease, are advised to stay away from fasting. If you have type 2 diabetes, you can probably fast but under a doctor's supervision.

What side effects can occur when following a 16/8?

Common initial side effects include severe hunger, constipation, headaches, dizziness, heartburn, muscle cramps, tiredness, etc. Most side effects will disappear within a couple of weeks once your body adapts to fasting.

Can I chew gum while fasting?

Yes, the effect is so small that it wouldn't affect your fast much. So, if you need to do that to get you through a fast, by all means, go for it.

Chapter 12: The 30-Day Challenge

Now that you have understood every possible aspect related to intermittent fasting and are well equipped with all the needed knowledge to get started, challenge yourself to a 30-day intermittent fasting schedule. If you have never fasted in your life, you can start slow instead of the 16/8 fast. Gradually build up your hours as days go by and you get comfortable fasting.

You can even make use of the 'My Fitness Pal' app to count your macros and calories to help plan your menus and make better choices with your food.

Recipes for Your Intermittent Fasting Menu

The following recipes with their nutritional values give you the macro constituents, so it is easy for you to pick a recipe of your choice and include it in your menu.

1. Herb Garlic Chicken - Keto friendly

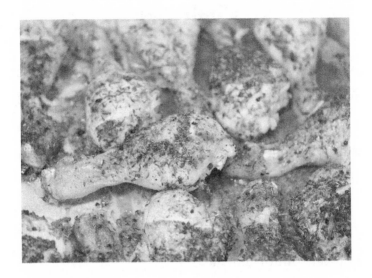

Ingredients

- Chicken drumsticks - 850gm
- Butter - 50 gm
- Juice of one lemon
- Salt and Pepper
- Crushed garlic cloves - 7
- Herbs of your choice - handful
- Olive oil - 2 tbsp

Directions

Wash and dry your chicken thoroughly. Sprinkle salt and pepper and rub into the meat. Preheat the oven to 450 degrees F. Prepare a baking tray by greasing it with butter. Place your chicken pieces, sprinkle the crushed garlic, lemon juice, herbs, and olive oil. Bake for 30 minutes until nicely golden brown.

Nutrition

Carbs - 3g Fats - 39g Proteins - 42g

2. Cauliflower Pancakes - Keto friendly

Ingredients

- Cauliflower - 500 gm
- Eggs - 3
- Small onion, grated - 1
- Salt and pepper
- Butter or vegetable oil for frying

Directions

Using a grater or a food processor grate your cauliflower finely. Take it in a bowl and add the remaining ingredients. On a hot skillet, make small pancakes out of the mixture about three inches wide until they start to bubble and flip, cooking the other side for less time. Serve hot.

Nutrition

Carbs - 5g Fats - 25g Proteins - 7g

3. Cheese and Jalapeno Meatballs - Keto friendly

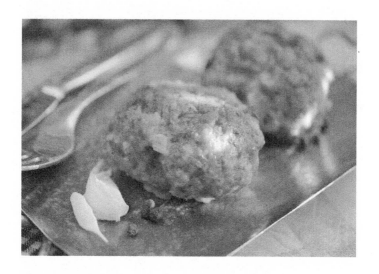

Ingredients

- Ground beef - 600 gm
- Egg - 1
- Pickled jalapenos - 50 gm
- Cheddar cheese - 100 gm
- Chili powder - 1 tsp
- Salt and pepper
- Vegetable oil for frying

Directions

Mix the cheese, jalapenos, chili powder, salt and pepper in a bowl. Add the ground beef and the egg. Mix well and form balls from the mixture. Fry the balls for 15 minutes until crispy.

Nutrition

Carbs - 1g Fats - 42g Proteins - 51g

4. Roasted Chicken with Garlic Butter - Keto friendly

Ingredients

- Chicken legs - 4
- Olive oil - 3 tbsp
- Italian seasoning - 1 tbsp
- Salt and pepper
- Butter - 100 gm
- Garlic, crushed - 3

Directions

Marinate the chicken legs with all the dry ingredients and keep aside for half an hour. In a separate bowl, mix together butter, garlic, salt, and pepper. Preheat the oven to 400 degrees F. Bake the chicken legs for 45 minutes or until golden brown. Serve hot with garlic butter and a favorite side of steamed veggies.

Nutrition

Carbs - 9g Fats - 60g Proteins - 28g

5. Cheesy Herb Omelet - Keto friendly

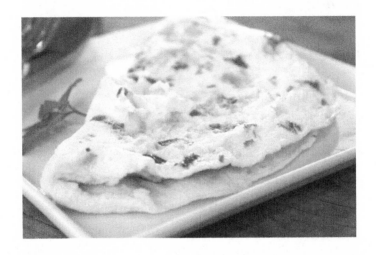

Ingredients

- Eggs - 6
- Cheddar cheese - 150gm
- Butter - 50gm
- Herb mixture of your choice
- Salt and pepper

Directions

In a bowl whisk eggs until frothy. Fold in half of the cheese and salt and pepper. Heat a pan and add the butter. When the butter melts, add the eggs, and sprinkle the herb mixture and the remaining cheese. Let the eggs cook for a few minutes until almost done. Fold and serve immediately.

Nutrition

Carbs - 4g Fats - 80g Proteins - 40g

6. Creamy Cabbage - Keto friendly

Ingredients

- Green cabbage - 600gm
- Butter - 50gm
- Heavy whipping cream - 300gm
- Salt and pepper
- Fresh coriander for garnish

Directions

Finely slice or grate the cabbage. Heat a pan and melt the butter. Add the cabbage and cook until soft and lightly brown around the edges. Add the cream and continue to stir until the mixture thickens. Add salt and pepper and garnish with coriander.

Nutrition

Carbs - 8g Fats - 38g Proteins - 5g

7. Chicken Veggie Soup - Keto friendly

Ingredients

- Cooked and shredded chicken - 900 gm
- Chopped carrots - 1 cup
- Chopped onion - ½ cup
- Chopped celery - ½ cup
- Minced garlic cloves - 5
- Chicken broth - 2 cups
- Water - 3 cups
- Butter - 50 gm
- Salt and pepper

Directions

In a large soup pot, melt the butter and add the chopped vegetables and the garlic. Cook for two minutes and add the chicken. Stir for a minute and add the broth and water. Let it come to a boil. Adjust salt and pepper.

Nutrition

Carbs - 4g Fats - 40g Proteins - 33g

8. Ground Beef with Beans - Keto friendly

Ingredients

- Ground beef - 300gm
- Green beans - 200gm
- Butter - 100gm
- Salt and pepper

Directions

In a large skillet melt half the butter and add beef. Fry until almost done for around 25 minutes. Add salt and pepper. In the same pan, add more butter to a side and fry the beans. Add salt and pepper. Stir fry for two more minutes and serve warm.

Nutrition

Carbs - 5g Fats - 50g Proteins - 30g

9. *Spicy Deviled Eggs - Keto friendly*

Ingredients

- Hard boiled eggs - 6
- Chili paste - 1 tbsp
- Mayonnaise - 100 gm
- Salt to taste
- Paprika to taste (optional garnish)

Directions

Shell hard boiled eggs and cut in half. Remove yolks into a bowl and add chili paste, mayonnaise, and salt. Mix well and scoop back into the egg whites. Garnish with paprika. Enjoy!

Nutrition

Carbs - 1g Fats - 20g Proteins - 6g

10. *Cheese Crisps*

Ingredients

- Shredded cheddar cheese - 200 gm
- Pepper to taste

Directions

Preheat the oven to 400 degrees F. Line a baking sheet with parchment paper, add heaps of cheese and sprinkle pepper on top. Bake for eight minutes or until the cheese is golden and crisp.

Nutrition

Carbs - 2g Fats - 19g Proteins - 12g

11. Scrambled Chili Eggs

Ingredients

- Eggs - 3
- Chopped green chilies - 1 tbsp
- Chopped tomato - ½ cup
- Salt and pepper
- Olive oil - 2tsp

Directions

Whisk eggs with salt and pepper until frothy. Heat oil in a pan and add the chilies and tomatoes. Fry until soft. Pour in the eggs and scramble up. Serve hot.

Nutrition

Carbs - 8g Fats - 11g Proteins - 20g

12. Bean and Corn Salad

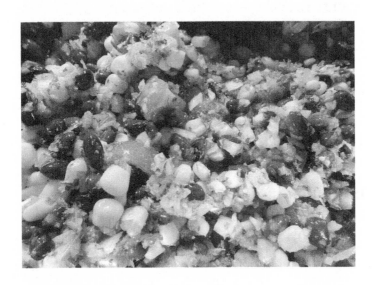

Ingredients

- Boiled chickpeas - 1 cup
- Boiled kidney beans - 1 cup
- Boiled corn - 1 cup
- Chopped tomato - ½ cup
- Chopped onion - 1 cup
- Chopped bell peppers - ½ cup
- Chopped green chilies - 1 tbsp

- Chopped coriander - ½ cup
- Salt and pepper
- Juice of one lemon

Directions

Toss all the ingredients together in a large bowl. Adjust seasoning to preference. Feel free to add more vegetables of your choice.

Nutrition

Carbs - 22g Fats - 1g Proteins - 34g

13. Macaroni and Beef

Ingredients

- Whole wheat macaroni - 2 cups
- Ground beef or lamb - 250gm
- Chopped onion - 1
- Pizza sauce - 1 cup
- Salt and pepper

Directions

In a large pan cook the beef and onions for around 30 minutes. In a separate vessel cook the macaroni until done and drain. In a separate bowl, mix the pizza sauce, macaroni, and cooked beef. Adjust salt and pepper. Serve hot.

Nutrition

Carbs - 28g Fats - 7g Proteins - 30g

14. Baked Balsamic Chicken

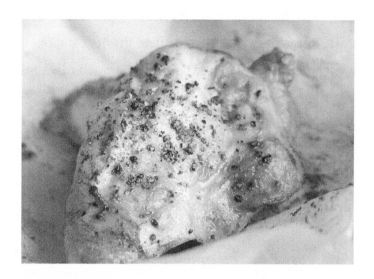

Ingredients

- Chicken breasts - 6
- Balsamic vinegar - ½ cup
- Brown sugar - 3 tbsp
- Chili powder - 1 tbsp
- Olive oil - 1 tbsp
- Salt and pepper
- Chopped parsley to garnish

Directions

Marinate the chicken with all the ingredients in a bowl. Refrigerate for 30 minutes. Preheat the oven to 375 degrees F. Coat a baking tray with olive oil and place the chicken. Bake until golden for 20 minutes. Garnish with parsley.

Nutrition

Carbs - 11g Fats - 9g Proteins - 28g

15. Cheesy Broccoli and Chicken

Ingredients

- Cooked and shredded chicken - 2 cups
- Blanched broccoli - 1 cup
- Shredded cheddar cheese - 1 cup
- Eggs - 2
- Low fat milk - ½ cup
- Salt and pepper

Directions

Preheat the oven to 375 degrees F. In a bowl whisk together the eggs, milk, salt, and pepper. In a large bowl mix together the chicken, broccoli, egg mixture, and half the cheese. Pour the mixture in a baking dish and sprinkle remaining cheese on top. Bake until the cheese is golden. Serve hot.

Nutrition

Carbs - 12g Fats - 8g Proteins - 20g

16. Chicken and Cheese Meatballs

Ingredients

- Ground chicken - 450gm
- Minced garlic cloves - 5
- Parmesan cheese - ¼ cup
- Italian seasoning - 1 tbsp
- Salt and pepper

Directions

Preheat the oven to 350 degrees F. Combine all the ingredients in a bowl and form walnut sized meatballs. Place these on a greased baking tray and bake for 15 minutes.

Nutrition

Carbs - 8g Fats - 6g Proteins - 30g

17. Cheesy Chili

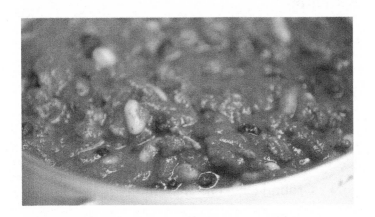

Ingredients

- Ground beef - 450gm
- Boiled kidney beans - 3 cups
- Chopped garlic - 1 tbsp
- Chopped onion - ½ cup
- Chili powder - 1 tbsp
- Shredded cheddar cheese - 1 cup
- Vegetable oil - 1 tbsp
- Salt to taste

Directions

Heat oil in a large pot and add the beef with onions. Cook for around 30 minutes till the beef is done. Add in garlic, kidney beans, salt, and chili powder. Let it simmer for 15 minutes. Adjust consistency by adding water. Serve piping hot garnished with cheese.

Nutrition

Carbs - 24g Fats - 14g Proteins - 32g

18. Lentil Cucumber Salad

Ingredients

- Boiled lentils - 2 cups
- Sweet corn - 1 cup
- Chopped cucumber - 1 cup
- Chopped tomatoes - 1 cup
- Tahini - 1 cup
- Balsamic vinegar - 2 tbsp
- Hot sauce - 1 tbsp
- Olive oil - 1 tbsp

- Salt and pepper

Directions

Mix all the wet ingredients with salt and pepper to form dressing. Toss all other ingredients in a large bowl and drizzle the dressing on top. Gently combine.

Nutrition

Carbs - 19g Fats - 13g Proteins - 27g

19. Chicken Quinoa Salad

Ingredients

- Cooked quinoa - 1 cup
- Cooked, shredded chicken - 1 cup
- Chopped tomatoes - ½ cup
- Chopped cucumber - ½ cup
- Chopped parsley - ½ cup
- Lemon juice - 1 tbsp
- Olive oil - 1 tbsp
- Minced garlic - 4
- Salt and pepper

Directions

Mix together lemon, olive oil, garlic, salt and pepper. In another bowl toss all the other ingredients. Pour the dressing and mix gently.

Nutrition

Carbs - 30g Fats - 14g Proteins - 31g

20. Almond Grape Smoothie

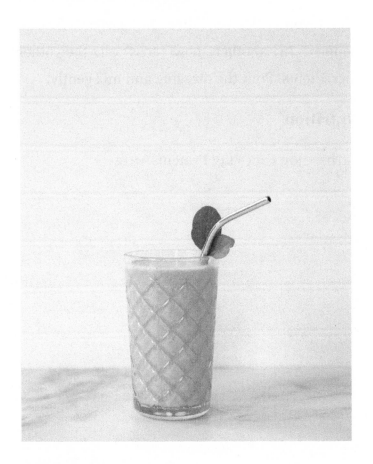

Ingredients

- Almond milk - 1 cup
- Green grapes - 20
- Peanut butter - 1 tbsp
- Yogurt - 1 cup

Directions

Add all the ingredients to a blender. Serve chilled.

Nutrition

Carbs - 11g Fats - 12g Proteins - 22g

21. Chocolate Banana Smoothie

Ingredients

- Chopped banana - 3
- Blanched almonds - 10
- Cocoa powder - 1 tbsp
- Milk - 2 cups
- Cooked quinoa - ½ cup

Directions

Blend all the ingredients together. Serve chilled.

Nutrition

Carbs - 18g Fats - 11g Proteins - 21g

22. Mixed Berry Smoothie

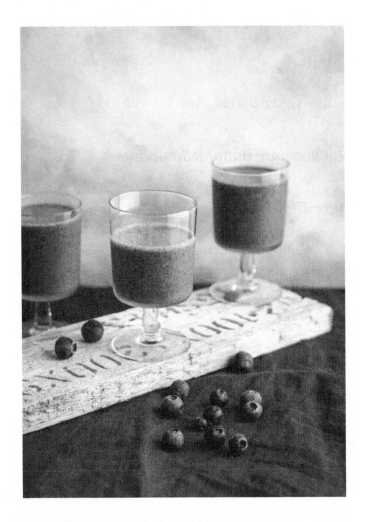

Ingredients

- Mixed berries of your choice - 3 cups
- Yogurt - 1 cup

- Honey - 1 tsp

Directions

Blend all the ingredients together. Serve chilled.

Nutrition

Carbs - 8g Fats - 7g Proteins - 19g

23. Soy Almond Smoothie

Ingredients

- Soy milk - ½ cup
- Almond milk - 1 cup
- Banana - 1
- Cooked oats - 1 cup
- Honey - 1 tsp

Directions

Blend all the ingredients together. Serve chilled.

Nutrition

Carbs - 15g Fats - 10g Proteins - 24g

You can calculate your required caloric intake for weight loss from the previous chapters. For a more involved and supportive weight loss journey feel free to post your progress, add questions, raise doubts and do a lot more in my Facebook group mentioned in the Intro.

Conclusion

Intermittent fasting is not just about weight loss, though weight loss is an essential part of the deal for most practitioners. But you really gain so much more from a 16/8 intermittent fasting schedule than just burning fat. This tool helps you practice any meaningful diet to the best of its ability without the disadvantages that come with fleeting fad diets.

Intermittent fasting is a great way to improve your brain function, sharpen your focus, enhance your memory and cognitive skills. It is an amazing lifestyle choice for any person at any stage of health. For someone who is looking to lose weight, build muscle or improve their overall health and quality of life, intermittent fasting is a great choice.

With its flexible schedules, non-rigid calories, and a menu of your choice, the 16/8 fasting plan lets you get in shape at your convenience with little extra effort.

If you are fed up with trying all the different diets, losing weight temporarily only to have it bounce back on you with vengeance, and are looking for something that actually gives you a way to achieve sustainable weight loss, then intermittent fasting is the way to go by all means. The 16/8 style of fasting, in particular, is the perfect choice for beginners.

Taking care of simple things like getting your fill during the eating window, drinking plenty of water to stay hydrated, using black coffee as means to curb hunger, and exercising regularly, can go a long way in making your intermittent fasting experience a success. Remember to start your fasts slowly and learn to listen to your body. The human body is complicated yet extremely intelligent machinery. It will adapt itself to the conditions around it and will signal you when it cannot handle it. If you are being too hard or harsh on your body, it will let you know. Learn to listen to these signs and adjust your schedules and meals according to what suits you best. Both in terms of what meals to eat and what exercises to include in your plan, give an ear to your body and understand its limitations. Remember to enjoy the process and truly feel your success all along your fasting journey by staying positive. Good luck!

References

Brown, J. (2018, November 28). *Is breakfast really the most important meal of the day?* BBC Future. https://www.bbc.com/future/article/2018 1126-is-breakfast-good-for-your-health

Cherney, S. W. and K. (2020, March 29). *11 Effects of Sleep Deprivation on Your Body.* Healthline. https://www.healthline.com/health/sleep-deprivation/effects-on-body#1

Moro, T., & Tinsley, G. (2016). *Effects of eight weeks of time-restricted feeding (16/8) on basal metabolism, maximal strength, body composition, inflammation, and cardiovascular risk factors in resistance-trained males.* Journal of Translational Medicine, 14(1). doi: 10.1186/s12967-016-1044-0

Young, A. (2020, January 29). *Want To Try Intermittent Fasting? This Method Is*

Science-Backed & Super Approachable. mbgfood. https://www.mindbodygreen.com/articles/16-8-intermittent-fasting-schedule

Made in the USA
Monee, IL
04 June 2020